# Spiral Slicer Recipes

## For Yummy and Easy Paleo, Gluten Free and Weight Loss Diets

**Sarah Sparrow**

PUBLISHED BY:
Sarah Sparrow
Copyright © 2014

*Disclaimer*

*The information contained in this book is for general information purposes only. The information is provided by the authors and while we endeavor to keep the information up to date and correct, we make no representations or warranties of any kind, express or implied, about the completeness, accuracy, reliability, suitability or availability with respect to the book or the information, products, services, or related graphics contained in the book for any purpose. Any reliance you place on such information is therefore strictly at your own risk.*

# Table of Contents

Introduction .......................................................................... 5

All Raw Dishes ..................................................................... 6

Nutty Pasta Marinara ........................................................... 6

Raw Pasta Meatless Ragu ...................................................... 8

Raw Broccoli Pesto Noodles ................................................. 10

Walnut Pesto Noodle Salad ................................................. 12

Raw Curry Noodles 2 Ways ................................................. 13

Raw Daikon Mei Fun ........................................................... 15

Raw Pad Thai ...................................................................... 16

Yellow Coconut Curry Noodles ............................................ 17

Raw Tomato Tapenade Over Cucumber Pasta ....................... 19

Garlic Sesame Salad ............................................................ 22

Asian Ginger Salad ............................................................. 23

Apricot Sesame Salad .......................................................... 24

Cooked Dishes .................................................................... 26

Zucchini Noodle Tuna Salad ............................................... 26

Veggie Chili ....................................................................... 27

Garden Salsa Pasta ............................................................. 29

Fire Roasted Bruschetta Zucchini Pasta .............................. 30

Veggie Chow Mein .............................................................. 31

Cashew Noodles .................................................................. 32

Sweet and Sour Noodles ...................................................... 33

Asian Daikon Stir-Fry ......................................................... 34

*Mushroom Zucchini Noodle Soup* .......................................... *35*

*Salmon in Lemongrass Broth*................................................ *36*

*Daikon Duck Soup* ............................................................. *37*

*Daikon Noodle Pho* ............................................................ *38*

# Introduction

Spiral slicers have made a big impact on the way raw food enthusiasts, vegans, vegetarians, and health conscious cooks make their meals. If you wanted pasta, noodles, or thin slices, you once had to use an old-fashioned and sometimes dangerous mandolin; or have expert skills to make those tiny slices yourself with a an extra-sharp kitchen knife. And those kitchen tools still never made the grade if you wanted perfectly strong and tender noodles without the carbs, wheat, gluten or cooking.

But now, with a spiral slicer and this recipe book, you can take zucchinis, cucumbers and other root veggies and make delicious noodle, pasta and salad dishes all in a snap. Using a spiral slicer is easy and convenient. It keeps your calories down, your carbs low, and your nutrients high. Make losing weight and gaining health as easy as slice, mix, eat. That's it!

Spiral slice to your heart's desire and make magic when you make your meals.

# All Raw Dishes

## Nutty Pasta Marinara

Prep Time: 10 minutes
Servings: 2

INGREDIENTS
1/2 butternut squash
Cashew Ragu:
2 medium tomatoes
1/2 cup cashew butter (or almond butter)
1/4 onion
2 garlic cloves
2 - 3 fresh basil leaves
1/2 teaspoon dried oregano
Sea salt (to taste)
Ground black pepper (to taste)
Water

INSTRUCTIONS
- Cut butternut squash in half and peel. Remove seeds and run through spiral slicer. Sprinkle with salt and pepper, to taste, and transfer to serving dish.
- For Cashew Ragu, peel and chop onion and garlic. Chop tomatoes. Add to food processor or high-speed blender with cashew butter, oregano, and salt and pepper, to taste. Process until thick sauce comes together, about 30 - 60 seconds.
- Top butternut noodles with Cashew Ragu and serve.

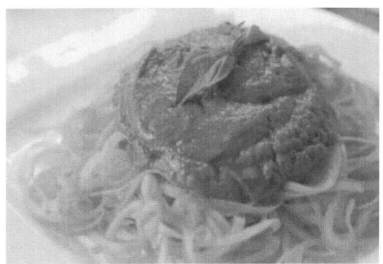

Photo by Saleeha Bamjee CC BY-SA 2.0

### Raw Pasta Meatless Ragu

Prep Time: 10 minutes
Soak Time: 2 hours
Servings: 1

INGREDIENTS
1 small zucchini
Ragu:
1/4 cup chopped walnuts (or 1/2 cup walnut halves)
2 small-medium tomatoes
2 tablespoons chopped onion
1 garlic clove
1/2 teaspoon sea salt
1/2 teaspoon ground black pepper
1/4 teaspoon dried basil
1/4 teaspoon dried oregano
Water

INSTRUCTIONS
- Chop walnuts and soak in enough water to cover for about 2 hours. Drain and rinse.
- For Ragu, peel and chop onion and garlic. Chop tomatoes. Add to food processor or high-speed blender with soaked walnuts, salt, pepper, basil and oregano. Pulse until chunky sauce comes together, about 30 seconds.
- Run zucchini through spiral slicer.   Sprinkle with salt and pepper. Transfer to serving dish. Top with Ragu and serve.

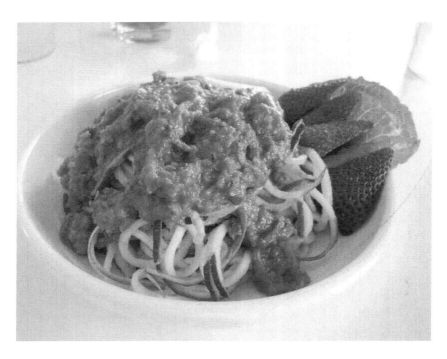

# Raw Broccoli Pesto Noodles

Prep Time: 5 minutes
Servings: 1

INGREDIENTS
1 small zucchini
Broccoli Pesto:
1/2 cup broccoli florets
1/4 cup fresh basil leaves (loosely packed)
2 tablespoons pine nuts
1/2 cup of tomatoes (soaked in water)
1 tablespoon nutritional yeast (optional)
1 - 2 tablespoons olive oil
1 large garlic clove
Sea salt (to taste)
Ground black pepper (to taste)

INSTRUCTIONS
- For Broccoli Pesto, peel garlic and add to food processor or high-speed blender with broccoli florets, tomatoes, basil leaves, pine nuts, olive oil, salt and pepper, to taste, and nutritional yeast (optional). Process until finely ground, about 30 - 60 seconds.
- Run zucchini through spiral slicer. Transfer to serving dish, top with the broccoli pesto and serve.

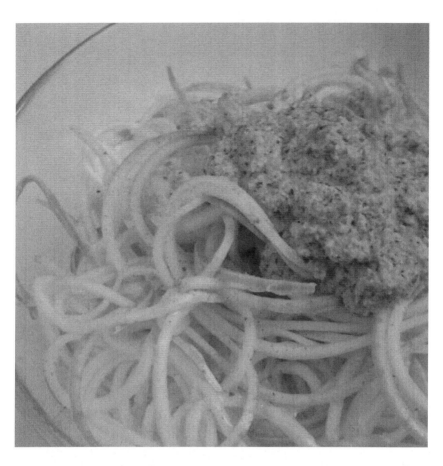

Photo by Lablascovegmenu CC BY 2.0

## Walnut Pesto Noodle Salad

Prep Time: 5 minutes
Servings: 1

INGREDIENTS
1 medium zucchini
1 small tomato
Walnut Pesto:
1/2 cup fresh basil leaves (tightly packed)
1/2 cup chopped walnuts (or 1 cup walnut halves)
2 tablespoons nutritional yeast
1 - 2 tablespoons olive oil
1 large garlic clove
Sea salt (to taste)
Ground black pepper (to taste)

INSTRUCTIONS
- For Walnut Pesto, peel garlic and add to food processor or high-speed blender with basil leaves, walnuts, olive oil, salt and pepper, to taste, and nutritional yeast. Process until finely ground, about 30 - 60 seconds.
- Run 2/3 zucchini through spiral slicer. Add to medium mixing bowl with Walnut Pesto. Toss with tongs to coat.
- Dice remaining 1/3 of zucchini, and tomato. Add to medium bowl and toss to combine.
- Transfer to serving dish and serve.

**Raw Curry Noodles 2 Ways**

Prep Time: 10 minutes
Servings: 2

INGREDIENTS
1 medium zucchini
1/4 cup chopped mushrooms
Green Curry:
1/4 cup fresh coconut meat (or soaked flaked coconut)
1/2 lemongrass stem
1/2 inch piece fresh ginger
1 garlic clove
1/4 lemon
1 teaspoon curry powder
Small handful fresh parsley
Sea salt (to taste)
Water
Red Curry:
2 tablespoons cashew butter (almond butter)
1/4 red bell pepper (or 2 tablespoons roasted red pepper)
2 teaspoons coconut aminos (or tamari or apple cider vinegar)
1/4 lemon
1 teaspoon curry powder
1/2 teaspoon ground turmeric
Pinch cayenne pepper
Sea salt (to taste)
Water

INSTRUCTIONS
- Run zucchini through spiral slicer. Split between two medium mixing bowls.
- For Green Curry, peel and chop garlic and ginger. Chop lemongrass stem. Add to food processor or high-speed blender with coconut, squeeze of lemon, curry powder, parsley and salt, to taste. Process with just enough water until smooth, about 30 – 60 seconds.
- Add to one mixing bowl and toss with zucchini noodles to combine. Transfer to serving dish.

- For Red Curry, add cashew butter, red pepper, coconut aminos, squeeze of lemon, curry powder, turmeric, cayenne pepper, and sea salt, to taste, to food processor or high speed blender. Process with just enough water until smooth, about 30 – 60 seconds.
- Add to remaining mixing bowl and toss with zucchini noodles to combine. Transfer to serving dish.
- Chop mushrooms. Sprinkle over Red Curry noodles and serve.

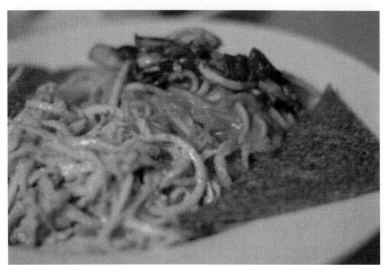

Photo by Marc Kjerland CC BY-SA 2.0

**Raw Daikon Mei Fun**

Prep Time: 10 minutes
Servings: 2

INGREDIENTS

1 large daikon radish
2 green onions (scallions)
1 carrot
1/4 cup cashew
Dressing:
2 tablespoon toasted sesame oil (or sesame oil or coconut oil)
1 1/2 tablespoons tamari (or coconut aminos or liquid aminos)
1/2 teaspoon soy sauce (or pure fish sauce)
1 teaspoon honey (or agave nectar)
1 garlic clove
1/4 inch piece fresh ginger
Sea salt (to taste)

INSTRUCTIONS
- Run daikon radish through spiral slicer. Run carrot through spiral slicer. Slice green onions. Add to medium mixing bowl.
- For Dressing, peel and chop garlic and ginger. Add to food processor or high-speed blender with sesame oil, tamari, soy sauce, honey and salt (to taste). Processes until emulsified, about 30 seconds.
- Add Dressing to mixing bowl and toss to coat.
- Transfer to serving dish. Sprinkle on cashew and serve.

**Raw Pad Thai**

Prep Time: 10 minutes
Servings: 2

INGREDIENTS
1 small zucchini
1 small carrot
1/2 purple cabbage
1/4 cup mung bean sprouts (optional)
Pad Thai Sauce:
2 tablespoons raw tahini
2 tablespoons raw cashew or almond butter
1 tablespoon lime juice (or lemon juice)
2 tablespoons raw apple cider vinegar (or tamari or coconut aminos)
1 tablespoon raw honey (or raw agave nectar)
1/2 large garlic clove
1/4 inch piece fresh ginger

INSTRUCTIONS
- Run zucchini through spiral slicer. Run carrot and 1/2 cabbage through spiral slicer. Add to medium mixing bowl with mung bean sprouts.
- For Pad Thai Sauce, peel ginger and garlic. Add to food processor or high-speed blender with tahini, cashew butter, lime juice, apple cider vinegar and honey. Process until smooth and creamy, about 1 minute.
- Add Pad Thai Sauce to mixing bowl and toss to coat.
- Transfer to serving dish and serve.

**Yellow Coconut Curry Noodles**

Prep Time: 10 minutes
Servings: 2

INGREDIENTS
1 medium-large zucchini
1/4 cup chopped pineapple
1 small carrot
1/4 red pepper
1/4 cup flaked or shredded coconut
Coconut Curry Sauce:
1/2 cup fresh coconut
1/2 lemon
2 garlic cloves
1 inch piece fresh ginger
1 tablespoon ground curry powder
1 teaspoon ground turmeric
1 teaspoon sea salt
Water

INSTRUCTIONS
- Run zucchini and carrot through spiral slicer. Chop pineapple meat. Thinly slice red pepper. Add to medium mixing bowl.
- For Coconut Curry Sauce, peel and chop garlic and ginger. Add to food processor or high-speed blender with coconut, lemon juice, curry powder, turmeric and salt, to taste. Process with just enough water until smooth, about 30 - 60 seconds.
- Add to mixing bowl with flaked coconut and toss to coat.
- Transfer to serving dish and serve.

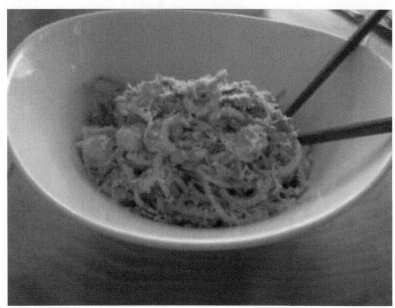

Photo by M Car CC BY-ND 2.0

# Raw Tomato Tapenade Over Cucumber Pasta

Prep Time: 10 minutes
Servings: 1

INGREDIENTS
1 small-medium cucumber
Walnut Parmesan:
1/4 cup walnuts
2 tablespoons nutritional yeast
Tomato Tapenade:
1/4 cup chopped mushrooms
1 small tomato
Small handful basil
Sea salt (to taste)
Ground black pepper (to taste)

INSTRUCTIONS
- Run cucumber through spiral slicer. Transfer to serving dish.
- For Tomato Tapenade, chop mushrooms and tomato. Chiffon (thinly slice) basil. Add over cucumber noodles and sprinkle with salt and pepper (to taste).
- For Walnut Parmesan, add walnuts and nutritional yeast to food processor or high-speed blender and process until finely ground, about 30 - 60 seconds.
- Sprinkle over dish and serve.

**Pasta Rustica**
Prep Time: 10 minutes
Servings: 1

INGREDIENTS
1 small zucchini
1/4 teaspoon dried thyme
1/4 teaspoon dried oregano
Sea salt (to taste)
Ground black pepper (to taste)
Marinara Rustica:
1/4 cup sundried tomatoes
1/4 roasted red peppers
4 dried apricots
1 large garlic clove
1/4 teaspoon dried thyme
1/4 teaspoon dried oregano
Sea salt (to taste)
Ground black pepper (to taste)
Water

INSTRUCTIONS
- Run zucchini through spiral slicer. Sprinkle with thyme, oregano and salt and pepper, to taste. Transfer to serving dish.
- For Rustica Marinara, peel garlic and add to food processor or high-speed blender with sundried tomatoes, roasted red peppers, thyme oregano, and salt and pepper, to taste. Process until thick sauce comes together, about 30 - 60 seconds.
- Top zucchini noodles with Marinara Rustica and serve.

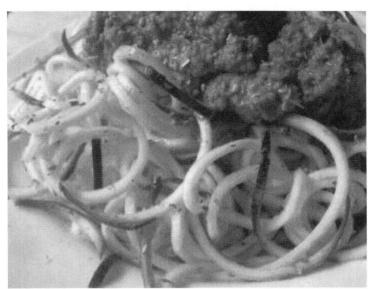

Photo by Lablascovegmenu CC BY 2.0

**Garlic Sesame Salad**

Prep Time: 5 minutes
Servings: 2

INGREDIENTS
1 small cucumber
1 small carrot
Small handful fresh parsley
Garlic Sesame Sauce:
1 tablespoons sesame oil
1 tablespoon soy sauce (or tamari or coconut aminos)
1 garlic clove
1/4 teaspoon sesame seeds (optional)

INSTRUCTIONS
- Run cucumber and carrot through spiral slicer. Add to medium mixing bowl.
- For Garlic Sesame Sauce, peel and mince garlic. Add to mixing bowl with sesame oil, soy sauce and sesame seeds (optional). Toss with tongs to coat.
- Transfer to serving dish and serve.

**Asian Ginger Salad**

Prep Time: 10 minutes
Servings: 2

INGREDIENTS
1/2 small purple cabbage
1/2 small green cabbage
1 carrot
1/3 cup walnuts
Ginger Dressing:
1/4 cup olive oil (or coconut, almond, walnut or sesame oil)
2 tablespoons balsamic vinegar (apple cider vinegar or rice vinegar)
1 tablespoon soy sauce (or tamari, liquid aminos or coconut aminos)
1 tablespoon honey (or agave nectar or coconut sugar)
1 garlic clove
2 inch piece fresh ginger
1/2 teaspoon toasted sesame oil (optional)
Sea salt (to taste)
Ground black pepper (to taste)

INSTRUCTIONS
- Run red and green cabbages through spiral slicer. Run carrot through spiral slicer. Add to large mixing bowl with walnuts.
- For Ginger Dressing, peel and chop ginger and garlic. Add to food processor or high-speed blender. Process until finely ground, about 30 seconds. Add olive oil, balsamic vinegar, soy sauce, honey, salt and pepper to taste, and sesame oil (optional.) Process until emulsified, about 30 seconds.
- Add Ginger Dressing to mixing bowl and toss to lightly coat.
- Transfer to serving dish and serve.

**Apricot Sesame Salad**

Prep Time: 10 minutes
Servings: 2

INGREDIENTS
1 heart of romaine
1 small carrot
1 small red onion
1/2 teaspoon black sesame seeds
Apricot Dressing:
1/4 cup toasted sesame oil (or sesame, coconut, almond, walnut or olive oil)
2 tablespoons apple cider vinegar (or rice vinegar)
2 tablespoons apricot preserves (or apricot jam)
1/2 inch piece fresh ginger (or 1 teaspoon candied ginger, minced)

INSTRUCTIONS
- Chop romaine lettuce and plate on serving dish.
- Run carrot through spiral slicer. Peel onion and run through spiral slicer. Add over plated romaine.
- For Apricot Dressing, peel and chop fresh ginger, if using. Or mince candied ginger. Add to food processor or high-speed blender and process until finely ground, about 30 seconds. Add sesame oil, vinegar, and apricot preserves. Process until emulsified, about 30 seconds.
- Drizzle Apricot Dressing over romaine, carrot and onion.
- Sprinkle on sesame seeds and serve.

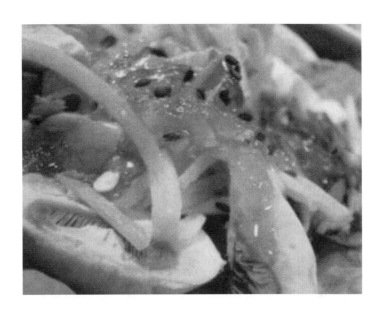

Photo by Vegan Feast Catering CC BY 2.0

# Cooked Dishes

## Zucchini Noodle Tuna Salad

Prep Time: 5 minutes
Servings: 1
INGREDIENTS
6 oz cooked tuna (chunk light or white albacore)
1 small-medium zucchini
1/2 small tomato
Small handful fresh parsley
1 - 2 teaspoons olive oil
Sea salt (to taste)
Ground black pepper (to taste)
INSTRUCTIONS

- Run zucchini through spiral slicer. Add to large mixing bowl.
- Chop tomato and parsley. Add to bowl with olive oil, salt and pepper, to taste. Toss with tongs.
- Rinse cooked tuna, if preferred, then drain. Add to bowl and toss until incorporated.
- Transfer to serving dish and serve.

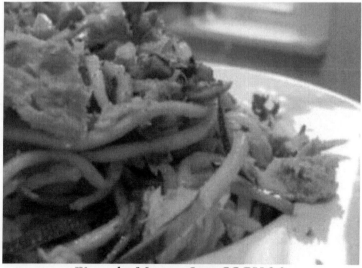

Photo by Mercury Jane CC BY 2.0
(Edited)

**Veggie Chili**

Prep Time: 10 minutes
Soak Time: 2 hours
Servings: 1

INGREDIENTS
1 medium zucchini
Veggie Chili:
1/3 cup chopped walnuts (or 2/3 cup walnut halves)
2 medium-large tomatoes
1/4 small onion
2 garlic cloves
1 tablespoon ground cumin
1 teaspoon chili powder
1 teaspoon sea salt
1 teaspoon ground black pepper
Water

INSTRUCTIONS
- Chop walnuts and soak in enough water to cover for about 2 hours. Drain and rinse.
- Heat small pan over medium heat. Dice 1/3 of zucchini and sprinkle with salt and pepper to taste, if preferred. Add to hot pan.
- For Veggie Chili, peel and chop onion and garlic. Chop tomatoes. Add to food processor or high-speed blender with soaked walnuts, salt, pepper, cumin and chili powder. Pulse until chunky sauce comes together, about 30 seconds.
- Add to zucchini and sauté about 2 minutes, until reduced and thickened. Remove from heat.
- Run remaining 2/3 of zucchini through spiral slicer.
- Transfer to serving dish. Top with Veggie Chili and serve.

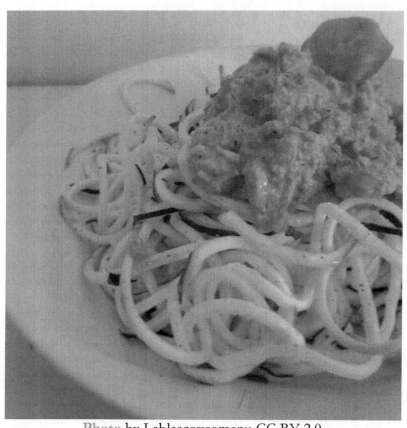

**Garden Salsa Pasta**

Prep Time: 10 minutes
Cook Time: 5 minutes
Servings: 1

INGREDIENTS
1 small-medium purple yam (purple sweet potato)
Garden Salsa:
1 medium tomato
1/2 small green pepper
1/4 small onion
1 garlic clove
1/4 jalapeño pepper (optional)
Small handful cilantro
1/2 lime
Sea salt (to taste)
Ground black pepper (to taste)

INSTRUCTIONS
- Bring medium pot of salt water to boil, then let gently simmer.
- Peel yam, if preferred. Run yam through spiral slicer. Add to simmering water and cook under lightly tender, about 5 minutes. Drain and transfer to serving dish.
- For Garden Salsa, peel onion, chop tomato and green pepper. Slice jalapeño (optional). Peel garlic. Add to food processor or high-speed blender with cilantro and squeeze of lime. Add salt and pepper, to taste. Pulse until chunky salsa forms, about 30 seconds.
- Top purple yam pasta with Garden Salsa and serve.

### Fire Roasted Bruschetta Zucchini Pasta

Prep Time: 5 minutes
Servings: 1

INGREDIENTS
1 small zucchini
Fire Roasted Bruschetta:
8 oz fire roasted tomatoes (whole or diced)
Small handful fresh basil leaves
2 garlic cloves
Sea salt (to taste)
Ground black pepper (to taste)

INSTRUCTIONS
- For Fire Roasted Bruschetta, peel and mince garlic. Chop or dice tomatoes. Chiffon (thinly slice) basil leaves. Add to small mixing bowl with salt and pepper, to taste. Mix to combine.
- Run zucchini through spiral slicer. Transfer to serving dish. Top with Fire Roasted Bruschetta and serve.

**Veggie Chow Mein**

Prep Time: 10 minutes
Cook Time: 10 minutes
Servings: 2

INGREDIENTS
1 medium zucchini
1/4 cup mushroom (button, Portobello, shitake, cremini, etc.)
1/2 small onion
1 small carrot
1 small celery stalk
1 scallion (green onion)
1/4 cup snow peas
2 garlic cloves
1/4 inch piece fresh ginger
2 tablespoons vegetable broth
Sea salt (to taste)
Ground black pepper (to taste)
1 - 2 tablespoons olive oil (or coconut oil)

INSTRUCTIONS
- Heat medium pan over medium-high heat. Add oil to hot pan.
- Peel onion, garlic and ginger. Mince garlic and ginger. Slice onions, carrot, celery and mushrooms. Thinly slice scallions.
- Add garlic and ginger to hot pan. Sauté about 30 seconds. Then add remaining veggies and sauté until lightly browned, about 5 minutes. Add vegetable broth and stir to combine.
- Run zucchini through spiral slicer.   Add to veggies and toss to combine. Let cook about 2 minutes. Season with salt and pepper.
- Transfer to serving dish and serve hot.

## Cashew Noodles

Prep Time: 5 minutes
Cook Time: 10 minutes
Servings: 1

INGREDIENTS
1 small zucchini
4 oz chicken breast (or tofu)
1 garlic clove
1/4 inch piece fresh ginger
Pinch fresh parsley
1 - 2 tablespoons olive oil (or coconut oil)
Cashew Sauce:
4 oz full-fat coconut milk
2 tablespoons cashew butter
2 tablespoons honey (or agave nectar)
1 teaspoon red curry paste (optional)
1/2 teaspoon apple cider vinegar (or white vinegar)

INSTRUCTIONS
- Heat medium pan over medium-high heat. Add oil to hot pan.
- Dice chicken or tofu. Add to hot pan and sauté about 2 minutes, until lightly browned.
- For Cashew Sauce, peel and mince garlic and ginger. Add to hot pan and sauté about 1 minute. Add coconut milk, cashew butter, honey, vinegar and curry paste (optional). Stir and let cook about 2 minutes. Do not burn.
- Run zucchini through spiral slicer.   Add to pan and toss to combine. Let cook about 2 minutes.
- Coarsely chop parsley and add to pan. Gently stir.
- Transfer to serving dish and serve hot.

**Sweet and Sour Noodles**

Prep Time: 10 minutes
Cook Time: 5 minutes
Servings: 2

INGREDIENTS
1 medium zucchini
1/2 cup green beans (chopped)
1 carrot
1/4 onion
1/4 cup walnut halves
Sweet and Sour Sauce:
1/4 cup pineapple juice
2 tablespoons ketchup
1 tablespoon apple cider vinegar (or white vinegar or rice vinegar)
1 teaspoon soy sauce

INSTRUCTIONS
- Heat medium pan over medium-high heat.
- Add walnuts to hot pan and toast about 2 minutes, stirring occasionally. Do not burn.
- For Sweet and Sour Sauce, add pineapple juice, ketchup, vinegar and soy sauce to hot pan and cook about 1 minute, stirring occasionally.
- Peel and chop onion. Chop green beans. Dice carrot. Add to pan and cook about 2 minutes.
- Run zucchini through spiral slicer. Add to hot pan and heat through about 1 minute.
- Transfer to serving dish and serve hot.

## Asian Daikon Stir-Fry

Prep Time: 10 minutes
Cook Time: 10 minutes
Servings: 2

INGREDIENTS
8 oz tofu (or chicken breast)
1 large daikon radish
2 cups broccoli (roughly chopped)
1/2 cup mung bean spouts
1/4 onion
1 carrot
2 garlic cloves
2 tablespoons soy sauce (or tamari or pure fish sauce)
Sea salt (to taste)
Ground black pepper (to taste)
Coconut oil (or peanut oil)

INSTRUCTIONS
- Heat medium pan over medium-high heat. Add oil to hot pan.
- Peel onion and garlic. Mince garlic. Slice onion. Chop carrot and broccoli. Chop tofu or chicken.
- Add garlic and tofu or chicken to hot pan. Sauté about 1 minute. Add onion, carrot and broccoli, and sauté until lightly browned, about 2 minutes. Remove and set aside.
- Run daikon radish through spiral slicer.
- Add daikon to hot pan with soy sauce and sauté about 2 minutes. Add browned veggies and protein back to pan with mung bean sprouts and stir to combine. Let heat through about 1 minute.
- Transfer to serving dish and serve hot.

# Mushroom Zucchini Noodle Soup

Prep Time: 15 minutes
Servings: 4

## INGREDIENTS
2 medium zucchinis
1 pint mushroom (button, Portobello, etc.)
2 quarts veggie or chicken broth (or stock)
Sea salt (to taste)
Ground black pepper (to taste)
Olive oil (or coconut oil)

## INSTRUCTIONS
- Heat medium pot over medium-high heat. Add oil to hot pot.
- Rinse and drain mushrooms. Dice 1 zucchini and mushrooms. Add to hot oiled pot with salt and pepper, to taste. Sauté about 1 - 2 minutes, until lightly browned.
- Add broth or stock to pot and increase burner to high heat. Bring to simmer then reduce to medium heat. Let simmer about 5 minutes.
- Run the other zucchini through spiral slicer. Add to hot broth and gently stir to combine. Let simmer another few minutes for softer noodles, if preferred.
- Transfer to serving dish and serve hot.

## Salmon in Lemongrass Broth

Prep Time: 10 minutes
Cook Time: 10 minutes
Servings: 1

INGREDIENTS
6 oz salmon fillet
1/2 daikon radish
1 small carrot
1/4 red onion
1/8 green cabbage
Sea salt (to taste)
Ground black pepper (to taste)
Coconut oil (or peanut oil)
Lemongrass Broth:
2 cups chicken broth (or veggie broth)
1 lemongrass stalk
2 - 3 basil leaves

INSTRUCTIONS
- Heat small pan over medium-high heat. Add oil to hot pan.
- Heat small pot over medium-high heat. Add broth.
- For Lemongrass Broth, smash lemon grass and split down center. Chiffon (thinly slice) basil. Add to broth and let simmer.
- Season salmon fillet with salt and pepper, to taste. Add to hot oiled pan and sear about 3 minutes on each side, until cooked through.
- Run daikon radish and carrot through spiral slicer. Chop thinly cabbage and onion. Add to hot broth and cook about 2 minutes.
- Remove lemongrass stalk and transfer Lemongrass Broth and noodles to serving dish. Top with salmon fillet and serve.

**Daikon Duck Soup**

Prep Time: 10 minutes
Cook Time: 10 minutes
Servings: 1

INGREDIENTS
2 cups chicken broth (or veggie broth)
4 oz duck breast fillet
1/2 daikon radish
1 small carrot
1/2 celery stalk
Sea salt (to taste)
Ground black pepper (to taste)
Coconut oil (or peanut oil)

INSTRUCTIONS
- Heat small pot over medium-high heat. Add oil to hot pot.
- Chop carrot and celery and add to hot pot. Sauté about 1 minute.
- Add duck breast to hot pot and sear 1 minute on each side.
- Remove duck breast fillet and slice. Add back to pot with broth and bring to simmer.
- Run daikon radish through spiral slicer. Add to hot broth and cook about 2 minutes.
- Transfer to serving dish and serve.

## Daikon Noodle Pho

Prep Time: 5 minutes
Cook Time: 10 minutes
Servings: 1

INGREDIENTS
2 cups chicken broth (or veggie broth)
1/2 daikon radish
1/2 scallion (green onion)
Large pinch fresh parsley
Sea salt (to taste)
Ground black pepper (to taste)

INSTRUCTIONS
- Heat small pot over medium-high heat. Add broth.
- Slice scallion and chop parsley Add to broth and let simmer.
- Run daikon radish through spiral slicer. Add to hot broth and cook about 2 minutes. Season with salt and pepper.
- Transfer to serving dish and serve.

Printed in Great Britain
by Amazon.co.uk, Ltd.,
Marston Gate.